THE AMAZING APPLE CIDER VINEGAR MIRACLE BOOK

Apple Cider Vinegar Secret Remedy for Health, Beauty and Home Cleansing

Lora C. Walter

Dedication

To all my readers

Acknowledgment

I want to say a huge thank you to my colleagues at "MySimpleHomeRemedies" for their invaluable support in making this book a success.

Table of Contents

INTRODUCTION

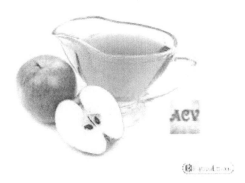

Apple Cider Vinegar provides some of the best cures to illness that afflict many. Germs and disease-causing organisms have evolved to stay with us, and they aren't going away soon. However, nature has given us what can keep sustaining our life form, and this time in the form of this precious liquid.

Apart from health, you can enhance your beauty with Apple Cider Vinegar. From sparkling teeth to lustrous hair and beautiful skin. It has been proven that those who use ACV rather than synthesized skincare products get more value for their money and avoid the long term effect of harsh chemicals on their skin.

Your home can also be made clean, safe, and neat without it putting a hole in your pocket. ACV is perfect as a stain remover and fabric softener, making it one of the best companions for laundry.

This book is written to expose you to the tried-and-trusted key benefits of Apple Cider Vinegar. It is structured in **three**

sections and subdivided into **chapters** that address each benefit.

Also, this book explains why ACV works for each benefit and teaches you how you can use ACV to achieve great results.

Chapter 1

WHAT IS APPLE CIDER VINEGAR

Apple Cider Vinegar has been with us for a very long time. Its legacy dated back to almost 8000 years ago, as much as the history books could cover. However, even around 6000 BCE, vessels loaded with barrels of Apple Cider Vinegar was found in China and Egypt.

There was also a record of Apple Cider Vinegar being used as condiment and preservative by the

Babylonians around 5000 B.C.E. More interestingly, it was postulated that they were the first to begin using Apple Cider Vinegar for herbs and as flavors for spice.

Apart from the uses of Vinegar in the kitchen, which had already been known for thousands of years back, Hippocrates first described the importance of Vinegar both in the prevention of illnesses and their treatment.

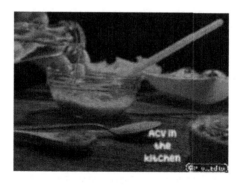

You may begin to wonder, what is this Apple Cider Vinegar with a wonderful history all about?

Well, Apple Cider Vinegar is the liquid obtained from the fermentation of Apple Cider. This means that if you allow Apple Cider to ferment long enough, the fluid obtained is what is called Apple Cider Vinegar. The whole process of fermentation converts the sugar in apples into alcohol and then into vinegar by the bacteria or yeast added into it.

Apple Cider Vinegar is acidic. A key component contributing to its acidity is Acetic Acid, just like other types of Vinegar.

Other essential components include:

- Lactic acid
- Citric Acid
- Malic acid
- And other fermentation bacteria.

Chapter 2

HOW TO PREPARE APPLE CIDER

As much as Apple Cider Vinegar is in different stores and supermarkets all around you, I still prefer the notion of preparing it yourself rather than spending money, which could be used for other things. Apple Cider Vinegar is easy to make, and there is a measure of trust regarding the content in your Vinegar bottle since you did it yourself.

Another advantage of preparing it yourself is that you won't have to bother if any chemical was added to the Vinegar in other to preserve it. You know the content in the bottle of Vinegar staring at you with the "Use-me-right-now" look.

I can't remember the last time I went to the supermarket to purchase a bottle of Apple Vinegar. I produce it myself in the comfort of my apartment.

Make your Vinegar

For making Vinegar, you can decide to use Peels and Cores or just stick to using chunks of apples. Each of these methods have their advantages and disadvantages

I prefer using the Peels and Cores because, here, nothing is wasted from the apples. The peels that otherwise could have been thrown away and allowed to decompose are being converted to useful products in the form of Vinegar. Cool!

Now let's get started with what you need in other to prepare yourself a great bottle of Apple Cider Vinegar.

Ingredients

For the preparation of your Apple Cider Vinegar, you will need;

- 3 cups of the fresh peels and cores from a healthy apple

- 2 tablespoon of genuine honey. You can also use sugar in place of honey if getting it proves difficult in your area

- 4 cups of clean water

The good thing about these ingredients is that they can all be got in any reputable supermarket around you. If you have them already in your refrigerator, then that's perfect. You could just start the preparation right away.

Tools

To make a unique vinegar, you will need certain tools to make the liquid come out clear and free from particles:

- A clean swatch of any clothing material or coffee filter

- A couple of rubber bands

- A clean air dried quart sized jar

- Fermentation weight

Of course, if you need more volume of Apple Cider Vinegar, you will need to get a bigger sized jar and more quantity of the ingredients.

Directions

- Bring out the quart sized jar and make sure it is clean. If not, wash it and air dry.

- Fill it the jar with the apple peels and cores. Make sure it doesn't pass ¾ mark on the jar. If you decide to use the whole apple method, then chop the apples into small bits and put them In the jar.

- Put clean water into the jar.

- Then pour in the raw honey and shake thoroughly. It takes time for raw honey to dissolve. If you use cane sugar, make sure you dissolve it in water first before you put in the jar.

- Make sure that the water in the jar covers the apples. I always like my apples submerged in the jar when I want to prepare my Vinegar.

- Place the jar on a fermentation weight to weigh the apples correctly. Although this step is not necessary and can be skipped. The advantage is that you do not want any apples exposed to air. It could form mould and corrupt the whole process. If the jar doesn't hold all the content, you can change jar or reduce the content in the jar.

- Now cover the jar with the clothing material you got and hold tight with the rubber band.

- Double-check if the jar is sealed correctly.

- Then store in a cool dark environment. Avoid putting it in a refrigerator. It is advisable to keep the covered jar in an environment with the standard room temperature (25 degrees centigrade).

- You are going to leave the mixture for about 3 weeks. If you begin using the vinegar before the 3rd completed weeks, it would not have fermented enough to be able to work effectively for whatever purpose you want to use it for. However, if you allow it to wait too long after the 3rd week, the acidic content would be more than the required, and it would become harmful for consumption.

- But you aren't going to just abandon your apple mix. Check it every day to ensure that the apples stay submerged and that there is no mold growing in the water.

- By the end of the 3rd week, you should start perceiving a fairly sweet smell. This is the time to remove the apple pieces. Leave the liquid in the jar.

- Now cover the jar and store it for another 3-4 weeks. Continue to stir the content and monitor daily.

- Observe the Apple Cider Vinegar until it has gotten to the tartness you want if it has within the stipulated 3-4 weeks period, then good. Just transfer the content from the jar into a clean container that can be sealed airtight.

- Your Apple Cider Vinegar is ready to use.

Section One

Apple Cider Vinegar for Good health

In this section, we would discuss all the benefits of Apple Cider Vinegar on your health.

There are numerous ways you could use ACV to promote good health and manage chronic illnesses.

This section is dedicated to providing answers to some of the significant challenges regarding health people spend money and other resources on.

Chapter 3

APPLE VINEGAR FOR WEIGHT LOSS

Consuming Apple Cider Vinegar is an excellent and harmless method of shedding that extra pound of flesh from your body. However, only a few people know this. A vast majority of big weight losers have gone through a rigorous routine to burn off their weight. Others use "special" drinks and drugs, which, of course, could have a dangerous effect on their overall health.

Why it works

Why does ACV impact so much on your health to make you lose weight in record time?

ACV reduces the total cholesterol in the body. A study done on rats, as published in the **British Journal of Nutrition,** stipulated that rats feed with Acetic acid in their diet –a component of Apple Cider Vinegar– had lower LDL, also known as bad cholesterol and higher levels of HDL compared to rats fed without.

Also, ACV suppresses your appetite. People who added weight rapidly knew that their hunger was their main culprit in pulling that stunt. With a reduction in how often you eat and the quantity of food consumed, you're less likely to gain weight. And if you're already on a course of weight gain, consuming ACV would be the best bet for you.

How to Use ACV

To enjoy the benefit of ACV on your weight loss program, it is required you take 1-2 tablespoons of Apple Cider Vinegar every day for up to 12 weeks. Take ACV before you eat any meal for the day, usually first thing in the morning. You will see a drop in your body weight, especially those fats around your belly.

However, some persons may not enjoy the taste of the Vinegar. If you are one of those, here is an excellent recipe to spice up your Apple Cider vinegar:

- **Mix with LEMON**: I recommend adding Lemon to your Vinegar when you want to use it for weight loss. This is because Lemon is known to help balance the pH of the liquid. Since you'll be taking Vinegar on an empty stomach, which is already acidic, lemon would neutralize the effect of the Vinegar in creating a less acidic environment.

Also. Lemon helps to reduce the amount of fat stored in your liver.

- **Mix with your FAVORITE JUICE:** Of course, ACV is one special liquid that allows you to mix it with any of your natural fruit juice. Whether you are an orange fan or you prefer a blend of strawberry, you can always get your Apple Cider Vinegar to taste better, precisely the way you like it.

Chapter 4

APPLE CIDER VINEGAR TO MANAGE DIABETES

The treatment of Diabetes, especially Type 2 diabetes or Non-Insulin Dependent Diabetes, is lifelong and sometimes very difficult to follow through. Most people do not keep up with their medications, and this worsens the overall outcome and course of the disease.

However, using Apple Cider Vinegar to control diabetes offers long term better effect and keeps the blood sugar level under control. The problem of type 2 diabetes lies in the fact that the body does not produce enough insulin for its usage and that the body cells are resistant to the small produced insulin.

Why it works

Apple Cider Vinegar controls diabetes in some ways:

1. ACV increases the uptake of glucose into the cells of your body, thus reducing the level of sugar in your blood.

2. Also, ACV makes your body more sensitive to the little insulin produced. That means that your

body would respond appropriately to insulin.

Above all, you are sure that with ACV as a regular feature of your diet, your medications would work more effectively.

How to use ACV

For Apple Cider Vinegar to properly keep your blood sugar level under control:

- Dilute 1-2 tablespoon of ACV in a glass of water.

- Make sure that you consume this mix before bedtime. That is the best time that ACV has in exerting its effect on your blood sugar level.

- Be careful not to consume the raw Apple Cider Vinegar.

- Continue for at least a week before you start seeing the effect.

- Do not also forget to seek your doctor's advice before you start this recipe. This is because some drugs may have an undesired effect when taken concurrently with Apple Cider Vinegar.

Other recipes

➢ **Cinnamon and ACV**

To prepare this recipe, you will need

- 1 tablespoon of ACV
- 1 tablespoon of stevia
- 1 tablespoon of finely ground Cinnamon

Then, make sure that you mix all ingredients properly in a clean pot.

The benefit of using Cinnamon is that it also helps to keep the blood sugar on a healthy level. Together with ACV, you're sure to get the maximum effect.

Take this mix twice daily for at least a week. Remember, it works best after meals and not on empty stomach.

➢ **Honey and ACV**

To prepare this unique recipe, you will need:

➢ 1 Tablespoon of ACV
➢ 1 teaspoon of genuine honey
➢ Half a cup of clean water

Add all the ingredients in a clean pot and mix it properly. You may need to mix all ingredients more prolonged than the other recipes mentioned above because of the viscosity of honey in this mix.

Take this drink twice a day.

Honey is unique because it helps to improve the taste of the Apple cider vinegar and helps strengthen your body immunity, which is needed for a person with diabetes.

Chapter 5

APPLE CIDER VINEGAR TO HELP ACID REFLUX

You may call it indigestion, the pain or burning sensation people feel in their chest sometimes when they consume spicy foods or foods that are rich in fatty acids. However, the pain might persist when you try to lie down or bend over.

That is called "Acid Reflux," and when symptoms of acid reflux, that is "Heart Burn" persists for long, it is called Gastro-esophageal Reflux

Disease (GERD). People with this problem are always feeling uncomfortable and usually assume different positions to alleviate the pain.

It is interesting to know that Apple Cider Vinegar has been used for centuries to treat this condition. The good thing is that you won't spend much trying to manage this condition using just ACV. You won't waste time trying to see a doctor.

Why it works

Part of the beneficial component of Apple is Pectin. Pectin is known to move substances such as food down along your digestive tract and help you stop feeling as if some is there that causes you discomfort

Besides, ACV helps to neutralize the acid content of your stomach. It is thought that the higher the acid production in your stomach, the more you tend to have reflux up your chest. That is why drugs that are used to treat this condition act by slowing down the production of acid in your stomach.

How to use ACV

The best way to use ACV to help your acid reflux is to include it in your salad dressing. Eating Salad helps improve your food digestion and relieve symptoms of indigestion. Thus, adding 1-2 teaspoons of ACV to it makes it more efficient.

Other Home Remedies for Reflux

For some individuals, using ACV can worsen their acid reflux. That is why you should try a little quantity of it to see if your body agrees with it. Whichever the case, here is a list of other remedies you can try for your acid reflux problems and symptom of heartburns.

➢ **Imbibe healthy eating practice.** This is very important if you want to overcome this health menace. Avoid very acidic foods. When eating, do not lie down. Also, avoid going to bed a few minutes after eating. Slow-and-steady eating is also encouraged. This would make sure that the food is correctly moved along your digestive system.

Also, avoid foods that can worsen reflux, such as:

1. Garlic
2. Alcohol
3. Spicy foods and mints.

These are but a few. Your doctor should make a list for you if you suffer from a severe kind of heartburn.

➢ **Keep away from Smoking:**
Several studies have linked smoking to acid reflux. This is because nicotine and most especially, tobacco has a relaxing effect on the muscles of the esophagus. Thus, making the stomach acids travel up easier.

Chapter 6

APPLE CIDER VINEGAR FOR ARTHRITIS

Arthritis is recognized as an age-related disease. However, some young individuals have been known to suffer from arthritis.

To simply put, Arthritis is a chronic inflammatory disorder of the bones and joints of the body such as the fingers, kneels, shoulders, hips, etc. characterized by pain, stiffness, and the inability to move these areas.

Why it works

There are many ways in which ACV helps to relieve Arthritic pain and improve symptoms. Some of them include:

➢ Apple Cider Vinegar raises the pH of the body. Arthritis thrives when the body pH is more acidic than necessary. What ACV does is to balance the body's pH when ingested.

➢ ACV also contains substances that stimulate the body enzymes to aid digestion and proper absorption of nutrients, which is required for the maintenance of healthy joints.

➤ Apple Cider Vinegar is rich in nutrients such as potassium, calcium, phosphorus, and magnesium. These nutrients help the body correct its deficiencies and thus helps to alleviate joint pains.

➤ Also, both magnesium and calcium are required for the proper growth, development, and maintenance of bones. Thus with the right amount of the essential nutrients coming from your apple cider vinegar drink, you can be sure that your arthritis would be appropriately managed.

How to use ACV

- You will need to take 1 teaspoon of raw apple cider vinegar first thing in the morning and also 1 teaspoon in the afternoon.

- If you do not like the taste of raw ACV, of course, not everyone does, you can add 1 teaspoon of honey. Stir it properly until the honey dissolves in the mix.

- If you do not have a bottle of genuine honey, you can mix your ACV with clean water. In that case, you will have to mix 1 teaspoon of ACV in ½ glass of water.

Chapter 7

APPLE CIDER VINEGAR FOR SORE THROAT

Your throat can become sore from excessive coughing or from a cold. Other times, it could be as a result of an infection. But whatever the cause of your sore throat, ACV provides a fast and better cure to your ailment.

Why it works

For one thing, ACV is known to possess excellent anti-microbial properties. Therefore, when ACV gets in contact with the sore areas of your throat, it can disinfect it and promote recovery. However, there are other properties of ACV that help fight against a sore throat.

They include:

➤ ACV contains Inulin, which is prebiotic. Inulin helps to increase the numbers of T cells in your body and helps to build your body immunity.

➤ It also functions as an expectorant. This means that it can loosen phlegm and therefore improves breathing and talking.

How to use ACV

There are many recipes that you can combine with ACV to give you a perfect cure for your sore throat. Otherwise, you can just proceed to use only ACV instead.

> **Diluted Cider Vinegar:**

To make this recipe, you will need

- A glass of warm water
- 1 tablespoon of ACV

Just mix the apple cider vinegar in the glass of water and stir gently. Then gargle several times a day with this mix. You can store the mix in a flask to keep it warm, or you can prepare a smaller quantity of the mix and use it immediately.

Other Remedies

➤ Cayenne pepper and ACV

To prepare this home remedy, you will need

- 3 teaspoon of raw honey
- 1 glass of clean, warm water
- 1 tablespoon of cayenne pepper
- 1 teaspoon of ACV

Get a clean bowl and pour all ingredients in it. Then mix them gently until you can get a uniform stir.

To use this remedy, you will gargle with it as often as possible. Then in between the gargling sessions, you will take in a little sip and swallow.

Most notably, do this immediately after you wake up early in the morning and as the last thing before going to bed.

> **Honey and ACV**

To prepare this remedy, you will need:

- 1 tablespoon of honey
- 1 tablespoon of ACV
- A glass of warm water

Mix all ingredients in the clean glass of warm water and drink once daily. I often recommend this remedy for a quick and perfect cure for a sore throat.

Honey also has antimicrobial properties, which, together with the

ACV, possess greater strength to fight off the bacteria causing you the sore throat. Honey also helps to relieve inflammation and pain.

Section 2

Apple Cider Vinegar for Beauty

In this section, we would discuss some of the most important uses of Apple Cider Vinegar for your overall beauty.

However, when we say beauty, we refer to the skin, hair, and teeth. This is so because those are the first things people notice when they see us.

Many people spend money trying to have the perfect skin complexion, glowing and dark hair, and sparkling teeth, fits that can be achieved without putting a hole in their pockets.

Chapter 8

APPLE CIDER VINEGAR FOR ECZEMA

Eczema is a common ailment affecting millions of people worldwide. It often results in dry, itchy and scaly skin. Eczema, also known as dermatitis, simply means inflammation of the skin. When we refer to Eczema in this context, we refer to a group of conditions that include: Atopic dermatitis, Dishydrotic Eczema, Contact dermatitis, amongst other forms.

If you suffer from this condition, you'll agree with me that you must have tried different forms of treatment to try and get it under control. However, there often would be relapses now and then even with the supposedly best forms of treatment.

I've seen many patients used some form of ointments, creams and gels and even drugs that only worsen their conditions. One fact I came to understand regarding Eczema is that going natural offers the best and lasting solutions, especially with atopic dermatitis, which, of course, as we know has genes that carry it. And when I say "Natural", I mean Apple Cider Vinegar.

Why it works

Research has shown that one way to improve symptoms of various skin disorders is to maintain the skin in its natural acidic pH. The skin is better managed at around a pH of 5.5. In other for skincare cosmetics to have any medicinal effect on the skin, most of them are prepared with this pH.

The more common alkaline soaps then to increase this pH and thus worsen the symptoms of dermatitis. However, with apple cider vinegar, the acidic pH of the skin is preserved. Studies have shown that patients who regularly use ACV on their skin have better recovery rates and more extended relapse period than people who use synthesized products for the skin condition.

Also, ACV has excellent anti-inflammatory properties, which can help manage the inflammation and infections that people with dermatitis often have. It heals and soothes broken skin, thus making it one of the best natural remedies available for Eczema.

How to use ACV

There're three ways you can use ACV to get maximum effect for your Eczema. Just choose any convenient one from the list and stick to it. In no time, your condition would resolve.

➢ **With A Warm Bath:** Just add a cup of ACV to your warm bath. Stir the mix, either in a big bucket or in your bathtub and allow for 15 minutes before you have your bath. Then rinse your body with cold water.

For quick effect, use ACV for your morning and night bath. However, because of the busy nature of some individuals, it's not feasible to wait for 15 minutes to allow the ACV mix properly. Then ACV should be used with a warm bath only at night when going to bed.

➢ **Use as a Hair Mask:** This is for people with scalp Eczema. Get ¼ cup of Sunflower oil and pour it in a bowl. Mix with 1 tablespoon of ACV.

Stir for 20 seconds to make sure that the ingredients mix properly. After you take a shower at night before bedtime, apply this remedy all over your scalp. The vinegar would help to retain the moisture on your hair, and this helps to avoid that flakiness and dryness on your scalp.

➢ **Use as a wet body wrap:** This method is better for those with Eczema around a defined area on their skin, rather than the extensive and scattered type of distribution. Just get a cup of warm water and add 1 tablespoon of ACV. Then get a clean cotton material or gauze and dip into the mix. Place this gauze around the affected area and hold firm with plaster. Allow it to sit for a while before you remove it.

However, before you try out this remedy for your Eczema, you should discuss it with your doctor. Some people may experience worsen of their Symptoms when they commence ACV therapy.

Chapter 9

APPLE CIDER VINEGAR FOR ACNE

Acne is one skin condition dreaded by many. Acne, they say, is a disorder of young people's skin. Actually, we are now seeing a couple of older individuals –past the acne age- still having acne. And for them, it's a long battle because they probably would have tried many skincare routines and treatments but to no avail.

Acne can be very difficult to treat. In fact, many products offer so many promises to end your acne. In the end, you only spend your cash to get them while they disappoint you.

Why bother about acne when you can send the zits away naturally with ACV?!

Why it works

Well, part of the cause of your acne is the bacteria that colonize your skin. In some ways, these bacteria end up multiplying because they see a very comfortable place for them with nourishment (sebum) on your skin. So one way to keep your acne under check is to kill these bacteria.

Now, this is where ACV comes into play. ACV has good anti-microbial properties that drastically reduce the numbers of these acne-causing germs. Specifically, ACV contains Lactic acid, Citric acid, and Succinic acid, which have been shown to reduce the growth of *Cutibacterium acnes* -formerly known as *Propionibacterium acnes*- the bacteria that cause acne.

Apart from killing these bacteria, the acids mentioned above also help to reduce inflammation –all those red bumps- on your skin and prevents acne scars from forming.

How to use ACV

Before you try out ACV on your skin for your acne, you should first carry out the patch test.

> **Patch test**: To do the patch test, mix 1 part ACV in a 2 parts water. Apply in a small area of your face and wait for about 15 minutes. Check to see if there is any sign of irritation around that place. If none, then you are good to proceed with the ACV therapy for your acne.

> If you have sensitive skin, you can further dilute the ACV in water using the 1 part Vinegar and 4 parts water ratio.

> Do not use your fingers to apply the mix on your face. Instead use a clean

cotton pad and dabble the liquid on the affected area. This is because your fingers may further introduce germs to your skin. Move-in a circular manner and cover all the affected areas.

➢ Wait for 20 minutes to make sure that the mixture dries on your skin. Then wash off with water and apply your skin moisturizer.

➢ Continue this routine twice a day for at least 3 weeks. You would see good improvement in your skin condition.

Chapter 10

APPLE CIDER VINEGAR FOR MOLE

Moles result when your skin cells – the Melanocytes- grow in a cluster, forming a kind of skin growth that looks round and darker than your complexion. Usually, the skin cells are supposed to spread throughout your skin. When the former occurs, your skin forms a little growth, which could be black or brown in appearance.

Moles commonly appear in the skin around childhood. Some remain after childhood, and it is thus common to find at least 10-40 moles during adulthood. However, the majority of these moles are harmless. So many people usually leave them unattended. If, for cosmetic reasons, you want to remove moles from your skin, Apple Cider Vinegar is usually the best tool to use.

Why ACV works

Acetic Acid, amongst other acids, is a vital component of ACV. This acid mainly carries out the effect of apple cider vinegar as a mole remover by burning the area of the skin that the mole grows on.

In addition, it has been found out that Malic acid and Tartaric acid, which are both present in ACV dissolve moles and remove them from your skin.

How to use ACV

➤ After you must have prepared your apple cider Vinegar or you decide to buy from your local supermarket, pour a little quantity in a clean cotton pad.

➤ Then use the pad to clean the area of your skin with moles.

➢ Do so in a circular manner and leave the pad on the skin for at least 1 hour.

➢ Continue this routine for a week to see results.

However, you should note that although most moles are harmless and would not cause you any problems, some can be dangerous. You should consult your dermatologist for such moles. Your dermatologist would offer you a definitive cure for such a mole.

Chapter 11

APPLE CIDER VINEGAR FOR SUNBURN

Sunburn may not be a major problem any longer because of the advent of anti-sunburn cosmetics and sunscreens. However, you can still come down with sunburn as in the following case scenarios:

- You could run out of sunscreens and forget to restock
- You may not also apply enough sunscreen for that outdoor activity

- Or the sunscreen you apply may not be the recommended for that particular weather.

Sunburn thus results when you spend time in the sun, long enough for it to start to damage your skin. It usually present with an area of redness and pain.

Anyway, no matter the scenario that exposes you to the UV effect of the sun, you can treat sunburn conveniently and effectively with Apple Cider Vinegar

Why it works

Many properties of the Apple Cider Vinegar make it a good cure for sunburn, whether severe or mild.

Firstly, ACV is anti-inflammatory. Thus, when applied on an area of skin that is inflamed, it reverses the process.

Secondly, ACV has a way of normalizing the skin pH. During the process of having a sunburn, there is an imbalance in the pH of the skin, which is tilted to favor inflammation and it signs of redness, pain and swelling.

How to use ACV

I will show you three methods in which you can use ACV to relieve sunburn. Choose any one of them that is suitable for you.

➢ **Spray Method:** In this method, you will need a spray can. Mix equal volumes of water and ACV in a bowl. Stir properly and pour some quantity into a spray can. Make sure that the can does not contain any other liquid. Close the can properly and store it in a cool environment. If you develop a sunburn, spray the content in the can onto the affected area and leave it for about 1 hour before you rinse with cold water.

➢ **Dab Method:** Get cotton clothing and dip it into a bowl containing apple cider vinegar mix. In the preparation of the ACV mix, make sure you use cold water. After, squeeze the cotton material and dap it onto the affected area of your skin.

➢ **Bath Method:** Add a little quantity of Apple Cider Vinegar into your bathing water and take a very cool bath with it. This would soothe your skin and make you feel better.

Also, after using Apple Cider Vinegar on your skin, you should apply a moisturizer to the affected area. If you have Aloe Vera gel or Coconut oil, the better.

Section 3

Apple Cider Vinegar for Home Cleansing and Cooking

In this section, we would discuss the crucial uses of Apple Cider Vinegar in the home, from cleaning and keeping everywhere tidy to its various use in cooking.

With ACV, you are sure to get results around your home that will surpass the effect of chemicals synthesized for that purpose.

Interestingly, our grandparents knew these ACV secrets. But it seems that it wasn't passed on to our generations or we failed to imbibe it in our way of life.

Whichever way, these secrets did not go down the grain.

‘

Chapter 12

APPLE CIDER VINEGAR AS DRAIN CLEANER

Drains can get real messy quickly. Worse, some stains are difficult to remove, even with the best of "stain remover." For others, their pipes become clogged and retain water for days making it smell foul. This problem can be taken care of by ACV.

How to use ACV

This remedy works best with Baking Soda. It helps to not only clean your drain but also to freshen it up.

- ➢ You will need to empty about ½- 1 cup of baking soda down your drain (the measurement should vary with the size of your kitchen drain).

- ➢ Then pour 1 cup of Apple Cider Vinegar.

- ➢ You would notice a kind of chemical reaction, like rigorous bubbling and fizzling in the drain.

- ➢ Just allow it to continue for the next 5-10 minutes.

➢ With hot water available, rinse your drain continuously for the next 30 seconds. This should be followed by pouring cold water along your pipe. This helps to push all the content in the drain through your plumbing system and to dissolve any clog that may have formed.

➢ Always remember that the longer the mixture sits inside your drain does not improve efficiency. Instead it may form more clogs which may be difficult to remove in the long run.

However, some clogs cannot be removed with ACV. For example, a small metal stuck in your drain would not dissolve by adding apple cider vinegar to it. In that scenario, you will have to make do with a "Drain snake" or a "Hanger" to pull out the clog.

Chapter 13

APPLE CIDER VINEGAR AS WEED KILLER

Taking care of weeds around the home could be stressful and tedious. Most people spend hundreds of dollars on herbicides to kill grasses around the compound, which, incidentally, are also dangerous to the environment. For them, the definitive solution to having no weed in their compound is making the floor tarred.

If you hate the idea of continually using the mower for grasses within your compound or using dangerous herbicides to kill the weed, Apple Cider Vinegar is the best bet for you.

Why it works

It is not rocket science that Apple Cider Vinegar serves as a natural herbicide and potent killer of weeds. This is because Acetic Acid, which is a vital component of ACV dries up and damages plant foliage.

Also, ACV increases the acidity of the soil to an intolerable level making it difficult for weeds to thrive on. Therefore, get your ACV ready and learn how to use it to kill weeds.

How to use ACV

To enjoy using your ACV as an herbicide, it's best if you can get a spray bottle.

➤ Pour undiluted Apple Cider Vinegar in a spray can and keep airtight.

➤ The type of foliage would determine the quantity of Apple Cider Vinegar used for it.

➤ For perennial foliage, you would need to spray it with more quantity of ACV. Make sure you cover the plant from the root to the leaves. You would also need to douse the soil with ACV. For these kinds of plants, you would also need to repeat the number of times you cover them with ACV.

➢ For the seasonal foliage, a single spray of ACV would sometimes suffice. However, you should pick out the yearly young leaf and spray them immediately.

➢ Whether the type of plants in your compound is the tougher perennial foliage or the new growth of seasonal foliage, the best time to spray these plants is a calm sunny day with no prediction of rainfall in the forecast. The ACV would quickly penetrate the plants and the soil without any possibility of dilution.

Chapter 14

APPLE CIDER VINEGAR FOR LAUNDRY

One of the best ways to use Apple Cider Vinegar at home is for Laundry. Apple Cider Vinegar is useful when it comes to softening hard water, pre-treating difficult stains, and boosting the efficacy of your regular home detergent. You can also use ACV to improve the brightness of your clothes' color.

Why it works

Apple Cider Vinegar works best for laundry because of its natural appeal, which is better for your overall health. Traditional fabric softeners are actually made with harmful chemicals that could affect the skin in the long run.

In addition, the fragrances from traditional detergents can cause allergic reactions, especially for susceptible individuals. For example, Asthmatic patients are being advised to avoid certain products. The aroma from Apple Cider Vinegar has not been known to trigger any allergic reactions.

The downside about the chemicals used to produce traditional fabric softeners is that they are made to remain in your fabrics even after you rinse them thoroughly with water.

Moreover, ACV contains antimicrobial properties, which makes it your best bet to get rid of odor-causing bacteria from your clothes.

How to use ACV

➤ **Blankets:** To get the best efficacy of ACV for your bedding, just add 2 cups of ACV to the water used to rinse the fabrics after washing with your regular detergent. You will observe that your blanket would get softer, and the soap would be thoroughly removed.

➢ **New Fabrics:** New fabrics are delicate and should be handled with care. Also, the chemicals used to make new clothes can irritate the skin if worn immediately after being removed from its pack. Therefore, soak all new clothes in a bucket of water mixes with 1 cup of vinegar. Then wash your clothes and rinse with clean water.

➢ **Special fabrics:** For silk, prepare a mixture of 2 tablespoon vinegar, ½ cup of mild detergent in a bucket of cold water and dip the material. Do not soak the silk material. Wash and rinse well and allow to dry.

Chapter 15

APPLE CIDER VINEGAR FOR HOME COOKING

Apple Cider Vinegar can serve as a functional kitchen companion if used judiciously. Here is a list of different things you can do with ACV in your kitchen you haven't tried yet:

To wash Vegetables and Fruit

Vegetables and fruits are often sprayed with pesticides. The residue of these chemicals can affect the taste of your cooking, especially when you want to use the fruits raw. Water simply cannot remove the pesticide from your vegetables even if you wash them thoroughly for hours. Apple Cider vinegar provides the best way in which you can clean your fruits thoroughly before eating them.

Also, water would not remove all the dirt and germs hidden in your fruits. Apple Cider Vinegar is known to possess antimicrobial properties. You can be sure that using apple cider vinegar to wash your fruits and vegetable would kill all the unseen germs.

How to use ACV

- Get a clean bowl and fill it with 4 cups of water and 1 part Vinegar. Actually, the quantity of cider wash is determined by the number of fruits you want to wash.

- Allow the fruits, let's say berries, in this case, to stay awhile in the cider mix. Usually, 5 minutes is the best time.

- Then wash them gently to make sure that there is no feeling of sand.

- Now transfer your fruits to a colander. You can also use the same Apple Cider Vinegar to wash many fruits in this manner.

- Finally, rinse with cold water and transfer to a clean storage container and keep in your refrigerator.

Use Vinegar in a Sauce

Vinegar is that missing ingredient you've not added to your sauce when the taste does not come out just right.

How to use ACV

- 1 or 2 tablespoons of Vinegar is perfect for your tomato sauce. Add it just before you finish your cooking.

- This is good because it helps to enhance all other flavors you have added to the sauce.

- However, avoid adding ACV too late to your sauce else your cooking begins to taste sappy like ACV.

- Add and stir ACV properly for it to blend perfectly.

Conclusion

Only a few has been said regarding the benefits of Apple Cider Vinegar; a lot still needs to be discovered. We hope that as science and medicine keep getting better, humanity can fully come to understand the power and miracle housed in this unique liquid.

For now, keep using ACV for what it is known for. This is because ACV is not and would never be the cure to every health problem existing in our today's world. Many ACV enthusiasts may try to overplay its importance and usefulness. If there is no scientific evidence to back up the fact that Apple Cider Vinegar works for a particular condition, you should avoid using ACV for it.

Luckily, ACV has not been found to cause any adverse effect on the body. Since it is purely natural and no addictive was introduced in its production, it is understandable. However, this does not mean that Acv should be used without restrictions. When necessary, it is always important to seek your doctor's opinion before using ACV as a second-line treatment option.

Thank you.

Lora C. Walter

About The Author

Lora C. Walter is a natural beauty enthusiast. She is well known for her works at "MySimpleHomeRemedies" where she writes articles about health, lifestyle and beauty.

Printed in Great Britain
by Amazon

26346675R00061